Fiber One Fun: 25 Quick, Healthy, and Delicious Fiber Recipes Ready in a Jiffy

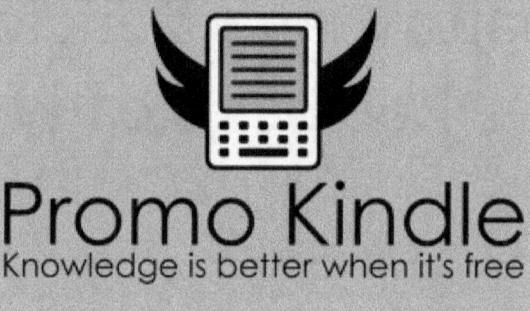

Disclaimer and Terms of Use: Effort has been made to ensure that the information in this book is accurate and complete, however, the author and the publisher do not warrant the accuracy of the information, text and graphics contained within the book due to the rapidly changing nature of science, research, known and unknown facts and Internet. The Author and the publisher do not hold any responsibility for errors, omissions or contrary interpretation of the subject matter herein. This book is presented solely for motivational and informational purposes only.

Table of Contents

Chocolate Peanut Butter

Ingredients:
- 1 bag chocolate chips
- ½ C peanut butter
- 3 ¾ C original bran cereal

Directions:

I.   Start with a cookie sheet lined with parchment paper
II.   Melt the chocolate chops and peanut butter in the microwave for about 1-1 ½ minutes until smooth
III.   Stir in cereal and drop by the spoonful on to the paper and refrigerate

Banana Bread

Ingredients:
- 2 C honey clusters
- ¾ C sugar
- ¼ C vegetable oil
- 1 C buttermilk
- 2 tsp. vanilla
- 1 egg
- 3 C flour
- 1 tsp. baking soda
- ¼ tsp. salt

Directions:

I.   Preheat your oven to 350 and grease bread pan
II.   Add cereal to Ziploc bag and crush cereal
III. In mixing bowl add everything together, cereal being last, spread throughout the pan
IV.   Bake for about an hour to an hour and 10 minutes
V.   Cool before serving, about 2 hours

Raisin Bran Muffins

Ingredients:
- 2 C Raisin Bran
- 1 ¼ C buttermilk
- ½ C raisins
- 1 tsp. vanilla
- ¼ C vegetable oil
- 1 egg
- 1 ¼ C flour
- ½ C brown sugar
- 1 tsp. baking soda
- ¼ salt

Directions:

I.   Preheat your oven to 400 degrees and grease your muffin tin
II.   Add cereal to Ziploc bag and seal, crush cereal, mix dry ingredients in one bowl
III. Add wet ingredients in another bowl, than combine the two bowls together
IV.   Divide batter amongst the muffin tins and bake for 18-20 minutes, let stand and cool

Honey Bars

Ingredients:
- 3 C honey clusters
- 1/4 C roasted nuts
- 1/2 C honey
- 1/4 C brown sugar
- 1 C dried apples
- 1/2 tsp. cinnamon
- 1/2 C peanut butter

Directions:

I.   Grease your baking dish
II. Add cereal to the Ziploc bag and crush cereal and set aside
III. Heat remaining ingredients and remove from heat, and pour over the crushed cereal and stir
IV. Add everything to your greased pan
V.   Press into pan and let sit in fridge for about an hour or so

Peanut Brownies

Ingredients:
- 1 tsp. cream cheese
- 1 tsp. peanut butter
- 1 fudge brownie
- 1 tsp. chocolate chips

Directions:

Blend first two ingredients and spread over bottom of brownie, sprinkle with chocolate chips and add top of brownie, making a brownie sandwich

Pop em' Brownies

Ingredients:
- 1 chocolate brownie (Fiber One)
- 1 T vanilla chips
- ½ tsp. sprinkles

Directions:

Add the brownie to a cake pop stick and roll in chips and sprinkles

Fiber One Chicken Nuggets

Ingredients:
- 1 C bran cereal
- 1/2 tsp. salt and pepper to taste
- 1/3 C mayo
- 1/3 C Dijon mustard
- 1/3 C honey
- 1 package chicken breast, strips

Directions:

I.   Preheat you oven to 400 degrees and spray cookie sheet
II.   Add cereal to bag, seal and smash cereal
III.   Mix mayo, mustard and honey, add this to chicken and toss cereal in as well, coating the chicken
IV.   Bake for 10 minutes, turn and bake

Cheesecake Bars

Ingredients:
- 1 Fiber One cookie
- 1 T cream cheese
- 1 tsp. powdered sugar
- 3 raspberries
- 1 tsp. powdered sugar

Directions:

I. Set your cookie on plate and add blended cream cheese and powdered sugar (well blended) to the top of your cookie

II. Garnish with raspberries on the top

Chicken and Avocado Salsa

Ingredients:
- ¾ C bran cereal
- 1 T ground cumin
- 1 tsp. lime peel
- ½ tsp. salt
- ¼ C buttermilk
- 4 chicken breast
- ½ tomato, chopped
- ½ avocado, chopped
- 1 T cilantro
- 1 tsp. jalapeno, chopped
- 1 tsp. lime juice
- salt and pepper to taste

Directions:

I.   Preheat oven to 400 degrees and spray cookie sheet
II.   Smash cereal in bag and mix with other garnishes, roll chicken in breading
III.   Bake for 20-25 minutes
IV.   Make salsa separately and serve with chicken

Baked Tilapia

Ingredients:

- 1 lb. tilapia
- 1 C Fiber One cereal
- 1 tsp. basil leaves
- salt and pepper to taste
- 1/4 C milk
- 1 T canola oil
- 1/3 C greek yogurt
- 1 tsp. horseradish
- 1 tsp. dijon mustard
- 1 chopped onion

Directions:

I. Preheat your oven to 400 degrees and spray cooking sheet
II. Add cereal to a bag and crush cereal
III. In bowl mix ingredients to make a coating for fish
IV. Bread the fish and bake for around 12-15 minutes

Parmesan Linguine

Ingredients:
- ½ C original Bran
- 2 T parmesan cheese
- ½ tsp. dried Italian seasoning
- ¼ tsp. garlic salt
- 1 egg white
- 2 tsp. milk
- 1 lb. chicken breasts, strips
- 1 T olive oil
- 6 oz. linguine
- 2 C vegetable pasta

Directions:

I. Preheat oven to 400 degrees, spray baking dish and smash cereal in a bag
II. Add everything to bag to bread chicken and bake for 20 minutes
III. Boil linguine and drain water
IV. Serve together, topped with pasta sauce

Turkey Burgers

Ingredients:

- 1 C bran cereal
- 1 lb. ground turkey
- 1/3 C chopped onion
- 1/4 C teriyaki sauce
- 1/2 tsp. ginger
- hamburger buns
- lettuce and tomato to garnish

Directions:

I. Crush cereal in baggy and add to turkey with other ingredients making patties
II. Grill over medium to high heat and serve with buns and garnish

Lemon Chili

Ingredients:
- 1 lb. fish filets
- 1 C bran cereal
- 1 tsp. lemon peel
- 1 tsp. chili powder
- salt and pepper to taste
- 1/4 C milk
- 2 T vegetable oil
- 1/3 C light mayo
- 1 T lemon juice
- 1/4 chili powder
- 1/4 C chopped cilantro

Directions:

I.   Preheat your oven to 450 and grease baking dish
II. Cut fish into slices
III. Crush cereal in bag and add remaining ingredients to bread fish
IV. Bake for 10-12 minutes

Snack Mix

Ingredients:
- 2 C bran cereal
- 2 C honey clusters
- 2 C honey cheerios
- 1 C raisins
- 1 C peanuts

Directions:

Add everything to Ziploc baggie and shake, serve

Green Tea

Ingredients:
- 6 C honey clusters
- 1 C cashews
- 1 C sesame sticks
- ¼ C brown sugar
- ½ C green tea
- 2 T honey
- 2 T vegetable oil
- ½ C dried mangos
- ½ C dried cranberries

Directions:

I.   Preheat oven to 200 and grease
II.   Mix dry ingredients together in bowl
III.   In saucepan mix sugars, honey, tea and oil, let simmer
IV.   Spread heated items for 30 minutes or so
V.   Stir items and bake a few more minutes
VI.   Let cool for about an hour

Bean and Veggie Dip

Ingredient:
- 1 C bran cereal
- 1 tomato, chopped
- 1 can black beans, drained
- 1 C water
- 2 T lemon juice
- ¼ C green onions
- 1 T Minced garlic
- salt and pepper to taste
- ½ tsp. cumin
- ½ tsp. cinnamon
- ½ tsp. chili powder
- ½ tsp. hot sauce
- 2 T cilantro
- 3 C fresh vegetables

Directions:

I.   Add everything but beans to food processor and blend until smooth
II.   Heat up 2-3 minutes stir in with blend and serve with vegetables

Pumpkin Trail Mix

Ingredients:
- 4 C bran cereal
- 1 C pretzel twists
- 1 C pumpkin seeds
- 1 C dried apricots
- 1/4 C chocolate chips

Directions:

Mix everything in a large bowl, transfer to plastic bag

Sweet Mix

Ingredients:
- 8 C popped popcorn
- 1 1/2 C bran cereal
- 1 oz. pretzel sticks
- 2 T chocolate chips
- 2 T salted peanuts

Directions:

Add everything to sealable bag or container and toss

Creamy Fruit Dessert

Ingredients:
- ½ C chopped strawberries
- ½ C green grapes
- 1 ½ tsp. chocolate chips
- ¼ C greek yogurt
- ¼ C bran cereal

Pumpkin Bars

Ingredients:
- 2 C bran
- ½ C oil
- ½ C orange juice
- 1 can pumpkin
- 2 eggs
- 1 ½ C flour
- 1 ½ C sugar
- 2 tsp. baking soda
- ½ tsp. ginger
- ¼ tsp. salt
- 1 C chopped walnuts
- 1 C powdered sugar
- 4 T orange juice

Directions:

I.   Preheat your oven to 350 degrees and grease your baking dish

II.   Add cereal to baggie, crushing cereal

III.   In bowl, add wet ingredients and blend, stir in cereal

IV.   Beat in other ingredients—everything but the walnuts

V.   Stir in walnuts

VI.   Spread batter in pan

VII.   Bake for 35-40 minutes

Cinnamon Apple Parfait

Ingredients:
- 1 C chopped apple
- ½ tsp. cinnamon
- ¼ C bran cereal
- 6 oz. vanilla yogurt
- 2 T whipped cream

Directions:

I.   Add cinnamon to bottom of bowl
II.   Layer the apples then cereal topped with yogurt and repeat

Crisp

Ingredients:
- 1/3 C sugar
- 1/4 C flour
- 2 bags blueberries
- 1 bag raspberries
- 1 1/2 C honey clusters
- 1/4 C chopped walnuts
- 2 T brown sugar
- 2 T butter

Directions:

I.   Preheat your oven to 375 degrees
II.   Mix together sugar and flour and berries
III.   Bake these uncovered for about 25 minutes
IV.   Crush cereal in bag and mix with remaining ingredients
V.   Sprinkle that mixture over baked berries and return to oven for another 20 to 25 minutes

Key Lime Pie

Ingredients
- 2 C bran cereal
- 1/4 C butter
- 1 T corn syrup
- 1 tsp. vanilla
- 2 T cold water
- 1 T lime juice
- 1 1/2 tsp. gelatin
- I package soft cream cheese
- 3 containers key lime yogurt
- 1/2 C frozen cool whip
- 2 tsp. lime

Directions:

I. Preheat your oven to 350 degrees, and crush cereal
II. In bowl mix crust together and press to the bottom of pie pan
III. Bake crust for about 10-12 minutes
IV. In pan, mix water and lime juice, add gelatin mix and let stand
V. Stir well, letting gelatin over low heat, and let stand for 2-3 minutes
VI. In separate bowl, beat your cream cheese, yogurt, and lime on low
VII. Fold in your cool whip
VIII. Refrigerate for around 2-3 hours

Turtle Brownies

Ingredients:

- 1 Fiber One brownie
- chocolate syrup
- 2-3 T honey bran cereal

Directions:

Layer brownie with the bran cereal followed by drizzled chocolate syrup

Raspberry Figs

Ingredients:
- Fig cookie
- 1 T raspberries
- Bran cereal

Directions:

Layer raspberry and cereal on top of fig cookies and serve

www.ingramcontent.com/pod-product-compliance
Lightning Source LLC
Chambersburg PA
CBHW070939290526
45795CB00003B/1084